BRONCHITIS DIET PLAN COOK BOOK

Recipes for a Healthy Bronchitis Diet That Really Works

REX LEWIS

Table of Contents

Introduction

The bronchial tubes, which are the airways that provide air to the lungs, are impacted by the inflammatory disease known as bronchitis. Acute and chronic bronchitis are the two main forms of the illness.

1. Serious Bronchitis:

• **Cause:** Viral infections, such the flu or the common cold, are usually to blame. Acute bronchitis can occasionally also result from bacterial infections.

• Symptoms include shortness of breath, exhaustion, coughing (frequently with mucus), and a low-grade temperature. It often lasts anything from a few days to several weeks.

• **Treatment:** Rest, fluids, and over-the-counter drugs can help relieve symptoms; this often goes away on its own. Antibiotics can be recommended if a bacterial infection is suspected, but they are ineffective against viral infections.

2. Chronic Bronchitis:

• **Cause:** Mostly linked to prolonged exposure to irritants such air pollution, cigarette smoke, dust, and chemicals at work.

- **Symptoms:** Recurrent respiratory infections, chest tightness, exhaustion, mucus-producing persistent cough, and weariness. Typically, symptoms persist for a minimum of three months throughout a period of two years.

- Management of symptoms and treating the underlying cause are the main goals of treatment. Giving up smoking is essential in situations involving tobacco smoke. To enhance lung function, doctors may recommend pulmonary rehabilitation along with medication.

Typical Qualities:

• **Danger Elements:**

• The main cause of chronic bronchitis is smoking.

• Environmental factors: Dust, odors, and pollution exposure.

• Immune system weakness: Makes a person more vulnerable to infections.

• **Diagnosis:** Based on medical history, physical examination, and occasionally diagnostic testing such pulmonary function tests or chest X-rays.

- **Prevention:** Reducing exposure to lung irritants and quitting smoking.

- Washing your hands frequently to avoid contracting viruses.

- **Complications:** Severe illnesses including chronic obstructive pulmonary disease (COPD) can develop from chronic bronchitis.

- **Symptomatic Relief:** For acute bronchitis, rest, fluids, and over-the-counter cough medications.

For chronic bronchitis, bronchodilators, steroids, and more oxygen are recommended.

It's vital to remember that seeking medical advice from a specialist is essential for an accurate diagnosis and suitable treatment if you suspect bronchitis or have chronic respiratory symptoms.

CHAPTER ONE
Diet is Crucial for Treating Bronchitis

The management of bronchitis is significantly influenced by food, since a nutritious and well-balanced diet can improve general respiratory health, lower inflammation, and boost the immune system. In order to effectively manage bronchitis, food is crucial in the following ways:

1. Hydration: Sustaining adequate hydration is crucial for preserving the respiratory tract's fluid content and aiding the body in removing mucus.

• Consuming enough fluids aids in preventing dehydration, which can exacerbate symptoms and impair the body's defenses against infections?

2.   Anti-Inflammatory   Foods: Reducing inflammation in the respiratory system can be achieved by including anti-inflammatory foods in the diet. Antioxidant-rich fruits and vegetables, like citrus fruits, leafy greens, and berries, are some examples.

• Omega-3 fatty acids are present in walnuts, flaxseeds, and seafood.

3. Vitamins and Minerals: Getting enough vitamins and minerals, particularly those that strengthen the immune system, can help the body heal. Some examples are as follows: Vitamin C: Found in bell peppers, citrus fruits, and strawberries.

• Spinach, carrots, and sweet potatoes are good sources of vitamin A.

• **Zinc:** Contains dairy, nuts, seeds, and meat.

4. Foods High in Protein:

• Protein is necessary for immune system maintenance and tissue repair. Tofu, salmon, beans, lentils, and poultry are examples of foods high in lean protein.

5. Steer Clear of Irritants: A few foods and drinks have the potential to aggravate bronchitis symptoms by irritating the respiratory system. One should steer clear of:

• **Coffee:** May lead to a dehydrated state.

• **Acidic or spicy foods:** May cause throat irritation.

Dairy products have been observed by certain individuals to elevate mucus production.

6. Sustaining a Healthy Weight:
Obesity puts stress on the respiratory system, which makes breathing more difficult. Maintaining a healthy weight and supporting lung function can be achieved with a balanced diet and frequent exercise.

7. Smaller, More Often Meals:
Eating smaller, more frequent meals rather than larger ones will assist reduce stomach distress and enhance comfort when breathing.

8. Consulting a Healthcare Professional:

• Dietary recommendations tailored to the specific needs of persons with underlying respiratory disorders or chronic bronchitis may be beneficial in certain situations. A customized dietary plan can be created with the assistance of a medical specialist, such as a pulmonologist or registered dietitian.

A balanced diet can help manage bronchitis, but it's important to incorporate dietary modifications within a comprehensive treatment plan that also includes rest, medicine, and other medical interventions. Always seek the opinion of a healthcare provider for specific recommendations based on your unique health situation.

Varieties of Bronchitis

Acute and chronic bronchitis are the two main forms of the illness. Their duration, causes, and characteristics are different.

The duration of acute bronchitis is usually brief, ranging from a few days to several weeks.

• **Cause:** Viral infections, such the flu or the common cold, are typically to blame. Acute bronchitis can occasionally also result from bacterial infections.

• Symptoms include shortness of breath, exhaustion, coughing (frequently with mucus), and a low-grade temperature. Acute bronchitis is a common respiratory ailment that frequently resolves on its own.

• **Treatment:** Rest, fluids, and over-the-counter drugs can help relieve symptoms; this often goes away on its own. Antibiotics can be recommended if a bacterial infection is suspected, but they are ineffective against viral infections.

2. Chronic Bronchitis:

• **Duration:** Persistent; symptoms must persist for a minimum of three months during a two-year period.

• **Cause:** Mostly linked to prolonged exposure to irritants such air pollution, cigarette smoke, dust, and chemicals at work.

• **Symptoms:** Recurrent respiratory infections, chest tightness, exhaustion, mucus-producing persistent cough, and weariness. One kind of chronic obstructive pulmonary illness is chronic bronchitis (COPD).

- **Intervention:** focuses on treating the underlying problem and managing the symptoms. Giving up smoking is essential in situations involving tobacco smoke. To enhance lung function, doctors may give drugs like steroids and bronchodilators. Supplemental oxygen and pulmonary rehabilitation could also be advised.

It's crucial to remember that, in contrast to acute bronchitis, which frequently resolves on its own, chronic bronchitis is a more serious, long-term illness that necessitates constant care and lifestyle modifications. Both forms of bronchitis cause inflammation of the bronchial passages, which results in symptoms including coughing up mucus and having trouble breathing. For an accurate diagnosis and suitable treatment, it's imperative to speak with a healthcare provider if you suspect bronchitis or have chronic respiratory symptoms.

CHAPTER TWO
Reasons and Signs

What Causes Bronchitis?

1. Acute Bronchitis:

• **Viral Infections:** Rhinovirus, influenza, and respiratory syncytial virus (RSV) infections are the most frequent causes of acute bronchitis.

• **Bacterial Infections:** Acute bronchitis can occasionally result from bacteria such as Bordetella pertussis or Mycoplasma pneumoniae.

• **Environmental Irritants:** Being around irritants such as dust, chemicals, smoke from tobacco, and air pollution can also cause irritation.

2. Sub-acute Bronchitis:

• **Smoking:** Prolonged exposure to cigarette smoke is the main contributing factor. The greatest risk factor for chronic bronchitis is this.

• **Environmental Factors:** Extended exposure to chemicals, dust, and air pollutants during work.

• **Recurrent Respiratory Infections:** Chronic bronchitis can be exacerbated by recurrent infections.

Common Bronchitis Symptoms:

1. Serious Bronchitis:

- **Cough:** Usually starts out dry and can eventually produce mucus.
- **Chest Pain:** Tightness or soreness in the chest area.
- **Fatigue:** Experiencing a lack of energy and fatigue.
- **Breathlessness:** Especially when exerting oneself.
- **Mild Fever:** Occasionally.

2. Chronic Bronchitis:

• **Persistent Cough:** A cough that is present on most days of the month for a minimum of two years in a row and lasts for three months or longer.

- Increased Mucus Production: Sputum production that is continuous or recurring.

- **Wheezing:** A squeaky or whistling sound made during inhalation.

- **Shortness of Breath:** A progressive breathing impairment.

- **Chest Tightness:** A tightness or pressure in the chest.

- **Recurrent Respiratory Infections:** As a result of impaired lung health.

General Signs and Symptoms of Both Types:

Breathing difficulties: Breathing can become more difficult, particularly while exerting yourself physically.

2. Cyanosis: A pale hue to the nails or lips as a result of insufficient blood oxygenation (more common in severe instances).

3. General Malaise: A generalized unease or discomfort.

4. Sore Throat: Pain or irritation in the throat, frequently connected to severe bronchitis.

It is significant to remember that symptoms might differ in severity and can be affected by personal factors including age, general health, and the existence of underlying medical disorders. Furthermore, chronic bronchitis necessitates continuing care and medical attention, although the symptoms of acute bronchitis frequently go away on their own. A medical professional's advice is crucial if you have persistent respiratory symptoms or suspect bronchitis in order to receive a proper diagnosis and course of therapy.

Dietary Influence on Bronchitis

When it comes to bronchitis, diet can play a big role in both managing and preventing the illness. The following are a few ways that diet may be involved:

1. Immune System Assistance: Vital vitamins and minerals can be obtained from a diet that is well-balanced and rich in a range of fruits, vegetables, whole grains, and lean meats. By bolstering the immune system, these nutrients assist the body's defenses against infections, particularly those that can cause bronchitis.

2. Anti-Inflammatory Foods: Including anti-inflammatory foods in your diet will help lessen respiratory tract inflammation. Antioxidant-rich foods like berries, citrus fruits, and leafy greens, along with omega-3 fatty acids from walnuts, flaxseeds, and fish, can help reduce inflammation.

3. Hydration: Keeping the respiratory tract wet requires drinking enough water. Sufficient hydration thins mucus, facilitating its removal from the respiratory system. Broths, herbal teas, and water are all healthy options for maintaining hydration.

4. Vitamins and Minerals: A number of nutrients are important for maintaining respiratory health. Citrus fruits and vegetables include vitamin C, which is well known for strengthening the immune system. Sweet potatoes, carrots, and spinach are good sources of vitamin A, which is necessary for the mucous membranes in the respiratory tract to stay healthy.

5. Protein Intake: Maintaining the immune system and repairing tissue both depend on consuming enough protein. Tofu, salmon, beans, lentils, and poultry are good sources of lean protein.

6. Steer Clear of Irritants: The respiratory tract might become irritated by certain foods and drinks. If caffeine, spicy meals, and acidic foods aggravate the symptoms of bronchitis, it might be best to avoid or consume them in moderation.

7. Sustaining a Healthy Weight: Obesity puts stress on the respiratory system, which makes breathing harder. A healthy weight can be maintained with a balanced diet and frequent exercise.

8. Individual Sensitivities: Certain dietary sensitivities may exist in some people, which may make respiratory symptoms worse. Dairy products have been seen by certain individuals to elevate mucus production. Recognizing and controlling one's own sensitivity can be useful.

It's crucial to remember that although maintaining a healthy diet will help, medical care is still necessary for treating bronchitis. A proper diagnosis and course of therapy, which may involve medication, rest, and other medical interventions, require speaking with a healthcare provider. Furthermore, individualized dietary recommendations based on individual health requirements may be advantageous for people with underlying respiratory disorders or chronic bronchitis.

CHAPTER THREE
Bronchitis Nutritional Guidelines

The goals of bronchitis nutritional guidelines are to enhance general respiratory health, lower inflammation, and strengthen the immune system. It's crucial to remember that the medical care recommended by a healthcare provider should not be substituted by these recommendations, but rather should be added to. **The Following Are Some General Dietary Guidelines For Bronchitis Sufferers:**

• **Remain Hydrated:** Sufficient hydration is essential to preserving the respiratory tract's fluid content. Herbal teas, broths, and water can all thin mucus and facilitate its removal from the respiratory system.

• Foods Rich in Antioxidants and Anti-Inflammatory Properties: Berries, citrus fruits, apples, and grapes are among the fruits that fall under this category.

• Carrots, sweet potatoes, broccoli, and leafy greens are examples of vegetables.

• **Omega-3 Fatty Acids:** Found in walnuts, flaxseeds, chia seeds, and fatty fish (mackerel, salmon).

- **Foods High in Vitamin C:**

Vitamin C strengthens the immune system. Add bell peppers, strawberries, kiwis, and citrus fruits (grapefruits, oranges) to your diet.

- **Sources of Vitamin A:** The health of mucous membranes depends on Vitamin A. Eat plenty of vitamin A-rich foods, like kale, sweet potatoes, carrots, and spinach.

- **Lean Proteins:**

 Protein is necessary for immunological response and tissue repair. Lean protein sources such as fish, chicken, beans, lentils, tofu, and low-fat dairy products should be included.

• **Steer Clear of Irritants:**

Restrict or stay away from foods and drinks that can irritate the respiratory system, particularly if they make symptoms worse. Caffeine, spicy food, and acidic food items may be examples of this.

• **Garlic and Onions:** These meals include substances that may strengthen the immune system and reduce inflammation. Include them in your meals for flavor and perhaps health advantages.

- **Probiotics:** Foods high in probiotics, such as kefir, yogurt with living cultures, and fermented foods like sauerkraut, may aid in promoting gut health, which is connected to immune system function in general.

- **Herbs and Spices:** Some herbs and spices, such as turmeric and ginger, have antioxidant and anti-inflammatory qualities. Think about incorporating them into meals or preparing calming drinks.

- Smaller, More Frequently Spaced Meals: o Eating more frequently spaced out meals can assist avoid overtaxing the digestive system and facilitate easier breathing.

- **Speak with a Medical Professional:**

Dietary recommendations tailored to the specific needs of individuals with underlying respiratory disorders or chronic bronchitis may be beneficial. Getting advice from a medical expert or licensed dietitian can assist develop a customized nutrition plan.

It's important to remember that these are only basic recommendations and that each person's dietary demands may differ. For individualized guidance based on your unique health situation, food choices, and any medications you may be taking, always seek the opinion of a healthcare provider.

Meal Preparation for the Flu

When it comes to bronchitis, meal planning should be centered on supplying the nutrients required to boost immunity, lessen inflammation, and preserve general health. Several nutrient-dense meals are included in this sample meal plan, which is as follows:

Breakfast:

1. Oatmeal with Berries:

- **Ingredients:** Rolled oats, water or milk (dairy or plant-based), a handful of mixed berries (strawberries, blueberries), and a drizzle of honey.

- **Benefits:** Berries supply vitamin C and antioxidants, and oats offer fiber.

2. Greek Yogurt Parfait:

- Made with Greek yogurt, granola, banana slices, and chia seeds as garnish.

• Health benefits include probiotics and protein from Greek yogurt, potassium from bananas, and fiber from granola.

3. Fruit Smoothie:

• **Ingredients:** Blend together a banana, a cup of almond milk, a handful of spinach, and a scoop of protein powder (if desired).

• **Benefits:** A vitamin, mineral, and hydration-rich smoothie full with nutrients.

4. Grilled Chicken Salad: Composed of grilled chicken breast, cucumbers, cherry tomatoes, mixed greens, and vinaigrette dressing.

- **Advantages:** Vitamins and antioxidants from a range of veggies, as well as lean protein from chicken.

5. Vegetable Soup:

• **Ingredients:** Carrots, celery, kale, and beans in a homemade or low-sodium store-bought soup.

- **Advantages:** veggies provide vitamins and minerals, hydration, and a calming effect from the heat.

6. Almond Butter and Banana Sandwich:

- **Ingredients:** sliced banana, whole-grain bread, and almond butter.

- **Advantages:** Rich in potassium from bananas, healthy fats from almond butter, and energy from complex carbs.

Supper Is

7. Baked fish with Quinoa.

- **Ingredients:** quinoa, steamed broccoli, lemon juice, **and** baked fish fillet.

- **Advantages:** broccoli provides extra vitamins, salmon provides omega-3 fatty acids, and quinoa provides protein.

8. Lentil and Sweet Potato Stew:

- **Ingredients:** lentils, tomatoes, onions, garlic, and vegetable broth.

- **Advantages:** Sweet potatoes provide beta-carotene, while lentils provide fiber and plant-based protein.

Evening Snack:

9. Turmeric Golden Milk:

- **Ingredients:** Ginger, turmeric, and a tiny bit of honey combined with warm milk (vegan or dairy).

- **Advantages:** Warmth can be calming before bed, and turmeric and ginger have anti-inflammatory qualities.

- **Hydration:** To stay hydrated and thin mucus, drink lots of water, herbal teas, or warm broths throughout the day.

- **General Advice:**

- **Steer clear of Irritants:** If caffeine, spicy meals, and acidic foods aggravate symptoms, limit or stay away from them.

- **Pay Attention to Your Body:** Modify serving sizes and dietary selections in accordance with personal comfort and hunger levels.

Recall that this meal plan is meant to serve as a broad reference; dietary restrictions and personal preferences should be considered. Always seek the opinion of a qualified dietitian or healthcare provider for individualized guidance based on your unique nutritional requirements and medical status.

CHAPTER FOUR
Importance of Regular Exercise

Frequent exercise has many positive effects on the body, mind, and emotions and is essential for preserving general health and wellbeing. The following are some major points underscoring the significance of consistent exercise:

Physical Condition:

1. Heart Health:

• Through enhancing blood circulation and cardiac power, exercise promotes cardiovascular health. It lowers blood pressure and lessens the risk of heart disease.

2. Controlling Weight:

• Engaging in regular physical activity helps maintain a healthy balance between caloric intake and expenditure while burning calories.

3. Strength of Muscles and Bones:

• Resistance training and weight-bearing activities enhance bone health by promoting muscle mass growth and lowering the risk of osteoporosis.

4. Enhanced Capacity for Respiration:

• Aerobic workouts improve respiratory health and lung

capacity, which improves oxygen exchange and lung health in general.

5. Improved Flexibility and Equilibrium:

• Particularly for older persons, stretching exercises and balance-enhancing activities lead to increased flexibility and a decreased risk of falls.

6. Enhanced Immune Response:

• Frequent moderate-intensity exercise has been associated with a boosted immune system, which lowers the risk of disease and enhances the body's defenses against infections.

Emotional and Mental Health:

1. Reducing Stress:

• The body's natural stress relievers, endorphins, are released when you exercise, which lifts your spirits and lessens worry and tension.

2. Better Quality Sleep:

• Studies have shown that regular exercise improves the quality of sleep by facilitating deeper and quicker sleep onset.

3. Mental Process:

• Cognitive function, such as memory, attention, and problem-solving abilities, is improved by exercise. Additionally, when people age, it might lessen their chance of dementia and cognitive decline.

4. Controlling Mood:

• Engaging in physical activity can help reduce anxiety and depressive symptoms, leading to a more stable and upbeat mood.

5. Enhanced Vitality:

• By enhancing general stamina and endurance, regular exercise helps to lower feelings of exhaustion and raise energy levels.

Benefits to Long-Term Health:

1. Prevention of Diseases:

• Regular exercise has been linked to a decreased chance of developing chronic illnesses, such as metabolic syndrome, type 2 diabetes, and several cancers.

2. Durability:

• Regular physical activity is associated with a longer life expectancy and improved quality of life as one ages.

3. Enhanced Body Image and Self-Esteem:

• By creating a good relationship with one's body and a sense of success, physical activity can help people feel better about their bodies and their self-esteem.

4. Relationship with Others:

• Exercise activities that are team- or group-based offer chances for social contact, which promotes a sense of support and community.

Suggestions:

• The World Health Organization (WHO) suggests engaging in

muscle-strengthening exercises two or more days a week in addition to 150 minutes of moderate-intensity aerobic activity or 75 minutes of vigorous-intensity exercise per week.

• It's critical to select activities based on personal interests, health problems, and fitness levels. Before beginning a new workout regimen, it is advisable to speak with a healthcare provider or fitness specialist, especially if you have any underlying health issues.

In conclusion, frequent exercise is essential to a healthy lifestyle since it provides a host of advantages for both physical and mental health, all of which enhance overall wellbeing.

Supplements and Herbal Remedies

Supplements and herbal therapies are frequently used in addition to conventional medicine to treat a variety of illnesses, including bronchitis. Even if there could be advantages to using certain herbs and supplements, you should proceed cautiously and speak with a healthcare provider before incorporating them into your routine. The following vitamins and herbal treatments are often thought to be effective for bronchitis:

Herbal Treatments:

1. Echinacea:

• Said to boost immunity and lessen the intensity and length of respiratory illnesses. It is frequently used to reduce cold symptoms and may be beneficial for acute bronchitis.

2. Ginger:

• Has antibacterial and anti-inflammatory qualities that may help ease sore throats and reduce coughing brought on by bronchitis.

3. Root Licorice:

• Licorice root, well-known for its expectorant and demulcent qualities, may aid in easing inflamed mucous membranes and encouraging the removal of mucus from the airways.

4. Thyme

• Has substances with antibacterial and expectorant qualities. Mucus can be released and coughing can be relieved with thyme tea or steam inhalation infused with thyme essential oil.

5. Mint pepper:

• Peppermint contains menthol, a chemical that cools the airways and may help reduce bronchitis-related cough and congestion.

6. Eucalyptus:

• Steam inhalation is a popular method of using eucalyptus oil to help clear respiratory congestion and facilitate easier breathing. It possesses bronchodilator and mucolytic qualities.

Addenda:

1. Vitamin C

• Renowned for strengthening the immune system, vitamin C may lessen the intensity and length of respiratory infections. Citrus fruits, berries, and supplements are common sources of it.

2. Zinc

• Boosts immunity and might lessen the intensity of cold symptoms. Supplements or lozenges containing zinc have occasionally been used to treat acute respiratory infections.

3. Vitamin D

• Contributes to immune system performance and may lower the incidence of respiratory infections. Sufficient exposure to sunlight and supplementation may be advantageous, particularly in the winter.

4. Probiotics:

• According to some study, probiotics, which encourage a balanced population of gut bacteria, may boost immunity and lower the risk of respiratory infections.

5. The Fatty Acids Omega-3:

• Omega-3 fatty acids, which are present in flaxseed and fish oils, have anti-inflammatory qualities and may aid in lowering airway inflammation.

Take Precautions:

• **Speak with a Healthcare Expert:** It's crucial to speak with a healthcare expert before utilizing herbal remedies or supplements for bronchitis, particularly if you're on medication or have underlying medical conditions.

• **Quality and Safety:** Make sure that supplements and herbal items come from reliable suppliers and are put through quality testing to confirm their safety and effectiveness.

• **Possible Interactions:** Certain vitamins and herbs have the potential to worsen pre-existing medical issues or interfere with prescriptions. Telling your healthcare practitioner about all the supplements you take is crucial.

• **Dosage and Duration:** Adhere to product labels or dosage guidelines from medical professionals. Avoid using some herbs or supplements for extended periods of time without a doctor's approval.

In conclusion, even though supplements and herbal medicines may be beneficial for bronchitis, it's important to use caution when using them and consult a healthcare provider for advice. By including these treatments into a thorough treatment plan that also includes dietary adjustments, lifestyle modifications, and traditional medical therapy, respiratory health can be optimally managed and supported.

How to Avoid Bronchitis Using Food and Lifestyle Changes

Making decisions that promote respiratory health and leading a healthy lifestyle are key to preventing bronchitis. Although total prevention of respiratory infections isn't always feasible, the following food and lifestyle choices may help lower the incidence of bronchitis:

Nutrition:

1. Rich in Nutrients Foods:

• Eat a well-balanced diet high in whole grains, fruits, vegetables, and lean meats to provide your immune system the vital nutrients it needs.

2. Drinking Plenty of Water

• Drink a lot of water and other liquids to be well hydrated. Drinking enough water aids in the body's removal of mucus and preserves the moisture content of the respiratory system.

3. Foods that Reduce Inflammation:

• To help lessen inflammation in the airways, include foods with anti-inflammatory qualities in your diet, such as leafy greens, berries, and fatty fish (high in omega-3 fatty acids).

4. Rich in Vitamin C Foods:

• Include foods high in vitamin C, which can support the health of the immune system, such as citrus fruits, strawberries, and bell peppers.

5. Probiotics:

• To support gut health and immunological function, eat foods high in probiotics, such as fermented foods, kefir, and yogurt with living cultures.

6. Restrict Irritants:

• Caffeine, spicy and acidic meals, and other irritants should be avoided or consumed in moderation since they might aggravate throat discomfort.

Way of life:

1. Quitting Smoking:

• Give up smoking or stay away from secondhand smoke. For respiratory disorders such as chronic bronchitis, smoking poses a serious risk.

2. Reduce Your Contact with Environmental Irritants:

• Reduce your exposure to dust, chemicals, and air pollution. When working in environments where respiratory irritants may be present, wear the proper protective gear.

3. Hand Sanitization:

• Maintain proper hand hygiene to lower your chance of contracting a virus that might cause acute bronchitis. Use hand sanitizer or routinely wash your hands with soap and water.

4. Frequent Workout:

• Get regular exercise because it strengthens the immune system and improves general health. Maintaining a healthy weight also helps with exercise, which eases the burden on the respiratory system.

5. Handling Stress:

• Engage in stress-relieving activities like yoga, meditation, or deep breathing. Prolonged stress can impair immunity and make a person more vulnerable to illnesses.

6. Sufficient Sleep:

• Make sure you get enough good sleep, as it's important for your immune system and general health.

7. Immunizations:

• Keep up with immunizations; if medical professionals advise it, get the annual influenza and pneumonia vaccines.

8. Steer Clear of Crowded Areas During Flu Season:

• To lower your chance of exposure, think about avoiding busy areas during flu season or other times when respiratory diseases are common.

9. Appropriate Ventilation

• To lower the concentration of indoor pollutants, make sure living and working areas have enough ventilation.

10. Frequent Medical Examinations:

• Make appointments for routine check-ups with medical professionals to keep an eye on your respiratory health, particularly if you have any chronic problems.

Keep in mind that these preventive steps are only recommendations and that each person's susceptibility to respiratory infections can differ. Seek guidance from medical professionals for tailored recommendations based on specific health problems and factors.

Conclusion

To sum up, bronchitis is a respiratory ailment that can have a substantial effect on people of all ages. It is characterized by inflammation of the bronchial tubes, which causes symptoms like coughing, soreness in the chest, and breathing difficulties. Although bacterial or viral infections can cause bronchitis, long-term exposure to irritants such as tobacco smoke or environmental pollution can also lead to the development of chronic bronchitis.

- Combining supportive care, lifestyle changes, and medication interventions is the approach taken to treat bronchitis. For bacterial infections, antibiotics may be recommended; for acute bronchitis, rest, fluids, and over-the-counter drugs can help relieve symptoms. Sustaining treatment for chronic bronchitis involves medicine, pulmonary rehabilitation, and quitting smoking.

• In order to effectively treat bronchitis, nutrition is essential. Anti-inflammatory foods, hydration beverages, and a well-balanced, nutrient-rich diet should all be included. Supplements and herbal treatments are frequently taken into consideration; however they should only be used sparingly and under a doctor's supervision.

Adopting a healthy lifestyle that includes quitting smoking, eating a balanced diet, getting regular exercise, and limiting exposure to respiratory irritants is key to preventing bronchitis. Vaccinations, adequate ventilation, and good hand cleanliness all help lower the risk of respiratory infections.

Healthcare specialists should always be consulted for an accurate diagnosis, customized treatment programs, and advice on lifestyle modifications. People can improve their general health and respiratory health by treating bronchitis holistically.

THE END